AROMATHERAPY

Simply for You

by Marion Del Gaudio Mak

Published by
Amberwood Publishing Ltd
Guildford England

ISBN 1-899308-10-5

Cover design by Howland Northover

Photography Mark Mak

Printed in Great Britain

CONTENTS

About the Author

Marion Del Gaudio Mak is a beauty therapist and aromatherapist currently lecturing at Southport College of Art and Technology. She is programme manager for beauty therapy, aromatherapy and sports therapy and is responsible for a range of courses incorporating, holistic therapy, reflexology, shiatsu, indian head massage and baby massage.

Marion has been an external examiner for the *International Health and Beauty Council* and is now an external assessor and verifier for them. She is also a member of *The Federation of Holistic Therapists* and *The International Federation of Aromatherapists.*

As a freelance consultant and trainer for beauty therapy and hairdressing salons her work often takes her overseas. She is regularly invited to speak to groups on the subject of aromatherapy.

Author's Foreword

As an experienced and qualified beauty therapist and aromatherapist currently lecturing in these subjects, I feel that everyone should have access to the benefits of aromatherapy.

I use essential oils in everyday life and for all purposes. I am well aware of the physiological and psychological effects that essential oils can have and want to ensure that others also share in the benefits, and experience perfect harmony and balance.

As a person who is totally committed to healthy living, natural health, skincare and therapies I feel that aromatherapy is a natural and beneficial way to aid healing; it is also a useful aid for treating minor ailments as well as a good alternative to commercial skin and haircare products.

I am often asked for advice on which essential oils may be used for various conditions and seem to spend a lot of time preparing information on essential oils and aromatherapy for people who would like to know simply how to use this popular therapy. This is why I have prepared this guide to using essential oils and aromatherapy. The recipes given are those which I formulate for my own use and are effective and pleasant to use. However, with a little bit of practice, you will soon be able to try out a variety of recipes to suit your individual tastes.

The information contained in this guide is straightforward and easy to follow. It should dispel many of the mysteries surrounding aromatherapy and enable everyone to benefit from the powers of essential oils in an easy to follow manner. Whilst I would always recommend visiting a professional, qualified aromatherapist, I realise that this is not always possible and that is why I have gathered this information to allow everyone to benefit from aromatherapy safely and simply.

Acknowledgements

I would like to thank Mum and Papa for my years at college, Concetta and Luigi for trying my Aromatherapy recipes, Mark for endless patience, encouragement and assistance, and Sophie for being my youngest Aromatherapy fan.

I would also like to thank Margaret and all my students, colleagues and special friends who have had so much faith in me.

Thanks also to June Crisp of Amberwood Limited for her enthusiasm.

Note to Reader

1 | Introduction to Aromatherapy

Aromatherapy is the use of aromatic oils which are derived from aromatic plant materials. These aromatic oils or essential oils are volatile and powerful substances, which are in effect, the "life force" of the plant. These tiny odoriferous molecules affect the mind and body and can bring about changes to the psychological and physical wellbeing.

In simpler terms, Aromatherapy is the use of essential oils to promote balance and harmony within mind and body! A natural and deliciously fragrant therapy for all the family.

ESSENTIAL OILS

Essential oils may be extracted from various sources of aromatic materials such as flowers, seeds, roots, barks and leaves. There are several methods of extracting these precious fragrant molecules from the source and they are as follows:

Distillation – aromatic plant materials are collected and placed into large vats, this is then steam distilled. When cooled the essential oil is separated leaving flower water.

Expression – essential oils are extracted by expressing or squeezing. This method is usually used for citrus oils where the peel or rind of the fruit is expressed to release the essential oils.

Solvent extraction – solvents are used to macerate delicate aromatic materials. The mixture is then treated to separate fragrant matter which is then distilled at low temperatures to produce the aromatic absolute.

2 | Essential Oil Purchasing and Storage

Before purchasing essential oils it is important to remember that the aromatic source from which essential oils are obtained is often extremely rare and precious and therefore the cost is often high. In order to ensure the purity of essential oils and therefore their therapeutic value, always purchase essential oils from a reputable supplier who is knowledgeable on the subject of essential oils and who can verify the source of origin of the oils. Allow price to be a good indicator also, as the more common the source of the essential oil, the cheaper the price and likewise, if the source of the essential oil is rare, the price will be higher. For example, expect to pay more for Jasmine than Lemon.

It is possible to purchase synthetically produced, or nature identical oils which will possess the same odour as a natural oil but may not have any therapeutic value. Beware of purchasing such a product.

Pure natural essential oils should be chosen to ensure that full benefits are gained from aromatherapy treatments. Remember that it is worth purchasing the very best that you can afford.

Essential oils are volatile, natural substances, and they are sensitive to light and heat. It is important, in order to maximise the life of essential oils, that they are stored in amber glass bottles with airtight lids to prevent oxidation and evaporation. Plastic bottles are unsuitable for essential oil storage as the essential oils will destroy the plastic and will themselves become tainted. Essential oils should be stored in a cool dark place avoiding any fluctuations in temperature. Ensure that the bottles are clearly labelled to indicate the contents, and ensure that children do not have access to essential oils.

The average shelf life of essential oils is approximately two years although citrus oils with the exception of Bergamot have a shorter life. Always replace the lid promptly after use to avoid oxidation.

Always purchase essential oils in small quantities and only as required in order to avoid wastage.

Essential oils are usually classified by their botanical species which is given in Latin.

For example: Lavender = Lavender angustifolia.

This helps to identify the correct source which allows essential oils to be chosen correctly. Always ask your supplier to check the botanical name if you require a particular essential oil for a specific action.

CAUTION

Although aromatherapy may be effective in treating many conditions safely and naturally, there are certain conditions which may not safely be treated as these require medical attention. It is always advisable to obtain professional medical treatment for serious conditions or whenever there is any doubt about the condition itself.

There are many conditions which will have contraindications or prevent the use of essential oils. As essential oils can cause the body to react in ways which may be harmful when certain conditions are present, it is important not to take any chances and always obtain medical consent if unsure.

You should seek medical permission before using essential oils if there is a history of illness or cancer in your family; also; if you are pregnant, diabetic, epileptic, or having medical treatments.

Remember that although essential oils are valuable healing aids, their action can be much slower than conventional cures and therefore if a condition is serious, professional help should be sought. Aromatherapy is a complementary therapy and must be treated as such.

If a condition worsens or fails to improve, medical help must be sought.

3 | How Essential Oils Work

Essential oils have Physiological and Psychological effects.

PHYSIOLOGICAL EFFECTS

Essential oils become effective when they enter the nasal cavity during inhalation and when applied to the skin they are absorbed into the blood stream. They are directed around the body to affect various organs according to the properties of the individual essential oils.

PSYCHOLOGICAL EFFECTS

Essential oils affect the mind when messages are sent as the essential oils enter the nasal cavity and stimulate the olfactory nerve which in turn initiates response from various areas of the brain to create reactions which deal with emotions and psychological wellbeing.

4 | Safety Precautions and Hazards

Essential oils must be treated with great respect as they are potent chemical substances and can be dangerous if not used correctly. Essential oils may be hazardous to the body and may result in reactions in certain individuals.

In order to check whether a sensitivity or allergic reaction will occur with essential oils, it is important to carry out a skin sensitivity test prior to using your chosen blend of essential oils.

A skin sensitivity test should be carried out twenty-four hours prior to using essential oils. It must also be remembered that an individual may develop an allergy at any time regardless of prior history.

If an essential oil is accidentally spilt onto the skin, the area should be flooded with a vegetable carrier oil which will dilute the effects of the essential oil. Neat essential oils must not be applied to the skin as they are too concentrated and will damage skin tissue.

Essential oils should be mixed in a vegetable carrier oil when used topically. Mineral oils and alcohol are not regarded as suitable carrier media for aromatherapy use. Water may be used when making up a compress or for hand and foot baths and must be agitated well in order to disperse the droplets of essential oil thoroughly.

For people with a history of skin sensitivity the following instructions should apply:

SKIN SENSITIVITY TEST
1. Blend required essential oils with carrier oil.
2. Wash and dry a small area of skin on the inner elbow.
3. Using a cotton bud, apply essential oil blend to the area.
4. Cover the area with a plaster and leave for 24–48 hours.
5. If irritation occurs, remove plaster.

6. If no adverse reactions are displayed, treatment may commence. If a reaction has developed this procedure must be repeated with other blends until a suitable combination is reached.

5 | Essential Oils

The following essential oils present risks of either toxicity, skin irritation or skin sensitisation, and are best avoided. They are considered unsuitable and under no circumstances should be used.

OILS UNSAFE FOR AROMATHERAPY USE

Almond (Bitter)	Prunus amygdalus
Boldo Leaf	Peumus boldus
Calamus	Acorus calamus
Camphor (Brown)	Cinnamomum camphora
Camphor (Yellow)	Cinnamomum camphora
Horseradish	Cochlearia armoracia
Jaborandi Leaf	Pilocarpus jaborandi
Mugwort	Artemesia vulgaris
Mustard	Brassica nigra
Pennyroyal (European)	Mentha pulegium
Rue	Ruta graveolens
Sassafras (Brazilian)	Sassafras albidum
Savin	Juniperus sabina
Southernwood	Artemesia abrotanum
Tansy	Tanacetum vulgare
Thuja (Cedarleaf)	Thuja occidentalis
Thuja Plicata	Thuja plicata
Wintergreen	Gaultheria procumbens
Wormseed	Chenopodium antheminticum
Wormwood	Artemesia absinthium

ESSENTIAL OILS WHICH ARE UNSAFE FOR USE ON THE SKIN

These essential oils must not be applied to the skin as they may cause serious damage or irritation. The essential oils in this group should be confined to use in pot pourri or environmental fragrance.

Cassia	Cinnamomum cassia
Clove Bud	Eugenia caryophyllata
Clove Leaf	Eugenia caryophyllata
Clove Stem	Eugenia caryophyllata
Cinnamon Bark	Cinnamon zeylanicum
Costus	Saussurea lappa
Elecampane	Inula helenium
Fennel (Bitter)	Foeniculum vulgare
Origanum	Origanum vulgare
Origanum (Spanish)	Thymus capitus
Pine (Dwarf)	Pinus pumilo
Savory (Summer)	Satureia hortensis

ESSENTIAL OILS WHICH MAY BE USED FOR AROMATHERAPY

The following essential oils are generally considered safe if used correctly. It should always be remembered that if used indiscriminately, all essential oils may be hazardous and that extreme caution should be exercised when choosing and using essential oils.

The following essential oils have been chosen for their value and versatility in treating a wide range of conditions. This is by no means a comprehensive list as there are many more essential oils available. You will discover that certain essential oils become firm favourites as you explore the delights of aromatherapy.

Basil	Ocimum basilicum
Benzoin	Styrax benzoin
Bergamot	Citrus bergamia
Black Pepper	Piper nigrum
Camomile (Roman)	Anthemis noblis
Cedarwood	Juniperus virginiana
Citronella	Cymbopogon nardus
Clary sage	Salvia sclarea
Cypress	Cupressus sempervirens
Cajuput	Melaleuca cajuputi
Cubeb	Piper cubeba
Eucalyptus	Eucalyptus globulus

Fennel (Sweet)	Foeniculum vulgare
Frankincense	Boswellia carteri
Geranium	Pelargonium graveolens
Grapefruit	Citrus paradisi
Ginger	Zingiber officinale
Ho Leaf	Cinnamomum camphora
Jasmine	Jasmium officinale
Juniper	Juniperus communis
Lavender	Lavender officinalis
Lemon.	Citrus limon
Lemongrass	Cymbopogon citratus
Lime	Citrus aurantifolia
Mandarin	Citrus reticulata.
Marjoram (Sweet)	Origanum marjorana
Melissa	Melissa officinalis
Myrrh	Commiphora myrrha
Neroli	Citrus aurantium
Orange (Sweet)	Citrus sinensis
Peppermint	Mentha piperita
Patchouli	Pogostemon patchouli
Petitgrain	Citrus bigaradia
Rose (Damask)	Rosa damascena
Rosemary	Rosemary officinalis
Sandalwood	Santalum album
Tea Tree	Melaleuca alternifolia
Vetiver	Vetiveria zizanioides
Ylang Ylang	Cananga odorata

ESSENTIAL OIL "NOTES"

For the purpose of blending, essential oils are classified into Top, Middle and Base notes. In order to ensure the best results from a blend it is important to choose an essential oil from each category.

Top Notes

These are essential oils which are stimulating to mind and body. They have sharp, crisp odours eg, Citrus, Eucalyptus. They last twenty-four hours before the odour evaporates.

Middle Notes

These are essential oils which affect bodily functions. They have flowery odours eg, Lavender, Marjoram, Geranium. They last two-three days before the odour evaporates.

Base Notes

These are essential oils which are soothing and calming. They have woody, resinous odours eg, Sandalwood, Myrrh. They last for one week before the odour evaporates.

If a base note is added to a top and a middle note it will "fix" or hold back the odour of the blend, allowing the properties of the chosen essential oils to remain effective for longer.

6 | Carrier Oils

Carrier oils are non-volatile substances which are extracted from the seeds of fruit and nuts. Carrier oils are used as a medium for essential oil application. A carrier oil should be chosen for its specific properties in relation to the type of skin or area of the body to which it will be applied. Some carrier oils have a distinct colour or odour and this should be taken into account when choosing in order to avoid heavy odours and staining of linen and clothing. Always purchase carrier oils in small amounts to ensure freshness, taking care that they are 'Cold Pressed', which means that they have been obtained from the natural properties. The pure, natural and unrefined carrier oils should be obtained from a reputable supplier who should be able to confirm the process by which the oil was obtained. Cold pressed carrier oils may turn slightly cloudy when stored at low temperatures, and, as previously explained, may possess a strong odour.

Carrier oils should always be stored in amber glass bottles with airtight lids as they may turn rancid if exposed to the air. Wheatgerm is the exception to this and is an excellent natural antioxidant. Wheatgerm may be added at 5% to all blends to prolong shelf life.

AVOCADO PEAR OIL – Dark green in colour. Excellent for dry, dehydrated skin and eczema. Use as a 10% dilution.

BORAGE SEED OIL – Pale yellow in colour. Suitable for psoriasis and prematurely aged skin. Use as a 10% dilution.

CORN OIL – Pale yellow in colour. Soothing for all skin types. May be used as 100% dilution.

EVENING PRIMROSE OIL – Pale yellow in colour, rich in gamma linoleic acid. Recommended for eczema, psoriasis, prematurely aged skin. Use as a 10% dilution.

SAFFLOWER OIL – Pale yellow in colour. May be used on all skin types. May be used as 100% dilution.

WHEATGERM OIL – Deep orange in colour. Suitable for eczema, psoriasis, dehydrated skin, stretchmarks. Use as a 10% dilution.

SWEET ALMOND OIL – Golden in colour. Excellent for dry, delicate skin, inflammation and itching. May be used as 100% dilution.

APRICOT KERNEL OIL – Pale gold in colour. Useful for sensitive, inflamed skin, ageing skin. May be used as 100% dilution.

GRAPESEED – Almost colourless. May be used for all skin types. May be used as 100% dilution.

HAZELNUT OIL – Golden in colour. Has an astringent action, good for oily skin and the body. May be used as 100% dilution.

JOJOBA – Pale golden, a liquid wax which mimics natural collagen. Excellent for all skin types especially oily, acne, and inflamed. Good for haircare. May be used as 100% dilution.

OLIVE OIL – Green in colour. Excellent for rheumatism, and skin cosmetics. May be used as a 10% dilution.

PEACH KERNEL – Delicate amber in colour. Particularly suitable for delicate, dry and dehydrated skin. May be used as a 100% dilution.

SESAME OIL – Dark golden in colour. Excellent for rheumatism, arthritis, and body care. May be used as a 10% dilution.

SUNFLOWER OIL – Pale yellow in colour. Useful for all skin types. May be used as 100% dilution.

7 | Blending Essential Oils

As all essential oils are potentially hazardous if used incorrectly, it is important to dilute them before use. Essential oils must never be applied directly to the skin, with the exceptions of Lavender and Tea Tree.

Always remember that essential oils are powerful natural substances and only small amounts are required.

As a general rule, proportions should never exceed 2½% and that for most applications this amount may be decreased. It is always best to use the lowest proportions possible.

EXAMPLES OF PROPORTIONS FOR BLENDING

Carrier Oil

200 drops of carrier oil, = 10ml carrier oil.
400 drops of carrier oil, = 20ml carrier oil.
1000 drops of carrier oil, = 50ml carrier oil.

Essential Oil

To 10ml carrier oil the maximum amount of drops of essential oil = 5 drops.
To 20ml carrier oil the maximum amount of drops of essential oil = 10 drops.
To 50ml carrier oil the maximum amount of drops of essential oil = 25 drops.

As an alternative carrier medium to vegetable oil, unperfumed, cleansing preparations, moisture creams and lotions, shampoos and conditioners may be used. However, the blending proportions remain the same and the maximum amount of essential oils must never be exceeded. Remember, also, that it is best to make up small batches of each blend in order to maintain the properties of the essential oil.

Proportions should be reduced according to your physical size and general condition. For example, a frail, elderly person will require less than a strong, physically fit person. Also, note that mood and general condition can greatly affect the way essential oils will influence a person.

For small children, blending proportions must not exceed 1%; babies require even smaller dosage, no more than ½%. ALWAYS USE EXTREME CAUTION.

8 | Methods of Using Essential Oils

There are many ways essential oils may be used every day to impart a sense of well being and balance. Using essential oils need not be a time consuming process. Aromatherapy is so simple and effective you will find yourself using various methods on a regular basis. Essential oils can be blended and carried with you to use wherever required.

BATHS – Add drops of essential oil to a bath full of warm water once steam has subsided. Use up to 6 drops of essential oil mixed into a teaspoon of full cream milk and agitate the water to aid dispersal of essential oils. Remain in the water for 15-20 minutes for maximum benefit. Alternatively, add essential oils to the carrier oil of your choice, massage into the skin before entering the bath, this will ensure that thorough penetration of essential oils takes place.

SHOWER – Add drops of essential oil to a washcloth or sponge which has been thoroughly wetted. Apply to the skin rubbing briskly whilst remaining under the shower.

FOOTBATH – Add up to 3 drops of essential oil to a footbath using the same method as for baths. Alternatively, essential oils may be added to an electric foot spa to make an effective foot treatment.

COMPRESS – Dip a pad of linen or cotton wool into a basin of water in which up to 3 drops of essential oil have been added. Apply to the affected area. Hot or cold water may be used according to the condition being treated.

VAPORISATION – Essential oils may be added to the vaporising light rings, diffusers, electric vaporising stones or onto a cotton wool ball or damp towel placed onto a radiator to diffuse the fragrant molecules into the atmosphere which can affect the physiological and psychological condition according to the essential oils chosen. This is a simple and effective way to use essential oils for treatment or environmental fragrancing.

STEAM INHALATION – Essential oils may be added to a bowl of hot water and inhaled under a towel. Essential oils may also be added to a facial steamer. Two drops of essential oils maximum.

MASSAGE – Add essential oils to a carrier oil or massage cream or lotion suitable for skin type and apply to the body with long, upward strokes. Use recommended dilution.

FACE MASKS – Add essential oil to natural clay, mixed to a paste with water. Apply to the face and remove when dry with warm water and sponges.

SKIN PREPARATIONS – Essential oils may be added to creams and lotions for skin care. Either add to bland commercial preparations or prepare your own, using natural ingredients. Skin toners may be prepared by adding essential oils to spring water and applying to the skin with a spray. It is advisable to choose lanolin-free preparations if skin sensitivity is apparent.

HAIR PREPARATIONS – Essential oils may be added to unperfumed shampoo and conditioner to beautify hair naturally. Deep conditioning preparations may be made using jojoba as a carrier to which the appropriate essential oils are added. Massage the blend well into the scalp and hair and leave for several hours or overnight. To remove the residue, apply shampoo neat to the hair, massage well before adding warm water. Apply weekly to maintain optimum condition of the hair and scalp.

AIR FRESHENERS/ENVIRONMENTAL FRAGRANCERS – Fill a plant spray with warm water, add essential oils and spray into the air. Air fresheners can be used to purify the air or to create subtle environmental fragrancing in a natural and pleasant way. Avoid spraying onto polished surfaces or delicate fabrics.

POT POURRI – Refresh fading pot pourri by adding one or two drops of essential oil and stirring. Create pot pourri fragrances to compliment the season and your mood. Make your own pot pourris by drying natural fragrant plant materials and scenting them with essential oils.

SCENTING LINEN – A few drops of the colourless or lighter essential oils may be added to the final rinsing water when laundering. Care must be taken to avoid staining and damage to delicate fabrics.

DIRECT APPLICATION – Lavender and Tea Tree are the only essential oils which may be safely applied directly to the skin. Useful for burns, cuts, bruises, spots etc.

INSECT REPELLENT – Apply essential oils neat to surfaces to repel insects. Essential oils may also be added to a water spray and sprayed as required.

HYGIENE IN THE HOME – As essential oils are powerful antiseptic and antibacterial agents, they are the natural choice for ensuring that the home is kept as germ-free as possible, and have the added bonus of fragrance.

Essential oils may added to hot water and detergent for wiping down work surfaces and floors etc. and are an effective and natural method for ensuring hygiene within the home. Essential oils are particularly useful in the kitchen and bathroom.

PROPERTIES OF ESSENTIAL OILS

Listed below are the essential oils together with some of their uses.

BASIL – Top/Middle Note. Uses – Antiseptic, digestive, memory stimulant, antidepressant.

BENZOIN – Base Note. Uses – Anti-inflammatory, antiseptic, expectorant, healing.

BERGAMOT – Top Note. Uses – Analgesic, antiseptic, antidepressant, diuretic. Avoid use prior to UVA exposure, as pigmentation and photosensitivity may occur.

BLACK PEPPER – Base Note. Uses – Poor circulation, rheumatism, catarrh, colds.

CEDARWOOD – Middle Note. Uses – Antiseptic, skin and haircare.

CITRONELLA – Middle Note. Uses – Insect repellent, fragrancing.

CHAMOMILE (ROMAN) – Middle Note. Uses – Analgesic, anti-septic, bactericidal, female reproductive system.

CLARY SAGE – Middle Note. Uses – Antidepressant, antiseptic, aphrodisiac, bactericidal, sedative, menstrual problems and pain, may be a powerful hallucinogenic.

CYPRESS – Top/Middle Note. Uses – Antirheumatic, antiseptic, deodorant, diuretic, astringent action, for broken capillaries and varicose veins.

CAJUPUT – Top Note. Uses – Antiseptic, expectorant, insecticide, for respiratory problems.

CUBEB – Middle Note. Uses – Catarrh, antiviral, respiratory problems, fragrancing.

EUCALYPTUS – Top Note. Uses – Analgesic, antiseptic, antiviral, decongestant, expectorant, stimulating oil.

FENNEL (SWEET) – Middle Note. Uses – Anti-inflammatory, antiseptic, diuretic, digestive.

FRANKINCENSE – Base Note. Uses – Anti-inflammatory, antiseptic, expectorant, sedative, ageing skin, wound healing.

GERANIUM – Middle Note. Uses – Antidepressant, anti-inflammatory, antiseptic, skincare.

GINGER – Top Note. Uses – Nausea, travel sickness, fragrancing.

GRAPEFRUIT – Top Note. Uses – Antiseptic, antitoxic, astringent, diuretic, cellulite, haircare.

HO LEAF – Top/Middle Note. Uses – Respiratory, catarrh, colds, flu, fragrancing.

JASMINE – Base Note. Uses – Antidepressant, anti-inflammatory, antiseptic, aphrodisiac, skincare, childbirth.

JUNIPER – Top Note. Uses – Antirheumatic, antiseptic, astringent, diuretic, skin and haircare.

LAVENDER – Middle Note. Uses – Analgesic, antiseptic, sedative, wound healing, general antiseptic use.

LEMON – Top Note. Uses – Antibacterial, antiseptic, antitoxic, diuretic, warts, viral infections.

LEMONGRASS – Top/Middle Note. Uses – Antiseptic, anti-depressant, bactericidal, insecticidal, stress relief, muscle toning.

LIME – Top Note. Uses – Antiseptic, antiviral, bactericidal.

MANDARIN – Top Note. Uses – Antiseptic, digestive, laxative, sedative, pregnancy.

MARJORAM – Middle Note. Uses – Analgesic, antiseptic, antiviral, diuretic, digestive, expectorant, sedative.

MELISSA – Middle Note. Uses – Calming, insect repellent, skin care.

MYRRH – Base Note. Uses – Anti-inflammatory, antiseptic, expectorant, skincare, wound healing.

NEROLI – Base Note. Uses – Antidepressant, antiseptic, aphrodisiac, nervous system.

ORANGE – Top Note. Uses – Antidepressant, antiseptic, digestive.

PATCHOULI – Base Note. Uses – Antiseptic, fungicidal, skin and haircare, wounds, ageing skin.

PEPPERMINT – Top/Middle Note. Uses – Digestive tonic, headaches, nausea.

PETITGRAIN – Middle Note. Uses – Antiseptic, skin and haircare, astringent.

ROSE – Base Note. Uses – Antidepressant, antiseptic, aphrodisiac, anti-toxic, sedative, skincare, female reproductive system.

ROSEMARY – Middle Note. Uses – Antirheumatic, antiseptic, astringent, digestive, diuretic, stimulating circulation, liver tonic.

SANDALWOOD – Base Note. Uses – Antidepressant, antiseptic, aphrodisiac, diuretic, sedative, expectorant, urinary problems, skincare.

TEA TREE – Top Note. Uses – Anti-inflammatory, antiseptic, anti-bacterial, antiviral, expectorant, strengthening the immune system, wound healing, thrush.

VETIVER – Base Note. Uses – Antiseptic, antitoxin, sedative, skincare, stress-related problems.

YLANG YLANG – Base Note. Uses – Antiseptic, aphrodisiac, sedative, skincare, haircare, (especially oily) stress-related problems.

9 | Ailments

The following is a list of ailments, and suggested essential oils which are effective in their treatment. As you become more familiar with essential oils and their effects you will also discover properties for yourself. Remember, however, that the effects of these essential oils may vary from one person to another in their efficacy and that sometimes patience is required as treatment times may vary also!

ACNE – Tea Tree, Lavender, Bergamot, Chamomile (Roman), Cajuput, Geranium, Patchouli.

ARTHRITIS – Chamomile (Roman), Lavender, Peppermint.

ACHING MUSCLES – Tea Tree, Lemongrass, Rosemary, Black Pepper.

ATHLETES FOOT – Tea Tree, Lavender.

BURNS – Lavender.

BOILS – Lavender, Tea Tree, Clary Sage.

BRUISES – Cypress, Lavender, Rosemary.

BROKEN CAPILLARIES – Lemon, Geranium.

CHILBLAINS – Lavender, Geranium.

CUTS AND ABRASIONS – Tea Tree, Lavender.

CELLULITE – Cypress, Geranium, Grapefruit, Juniper, Fennel.

CATARRH – Benzion, Eucalyptus, Cubeb, Sandalwood.

COLDS AND FLU – Benzion, Cubeb, Eucalyptus, Tea Tree, Rosemary, Black Pepper, Ho Leaf.

COLD SORE – Tea Tree, Bergamot, Lavender.

CONSTIPATION – Orange.

BITES AND STINGS – Tea Tree, Lavender, Basil.

DANDRUFF – Tea Tree, Cedarwood.

ECZEMA – Chamomile (Roman), Lavender.

FATIGUE – Geranium, Grapefruit, Mandarin, Vetiver.

FLATULENCE – Fennel, Mandarin, Petitgrain.

FLUID RETENTION – Fennel, Lemon, Cypress, Juniper.

HAIRCARE – Chamomile (Roman), Grapefruit, Geranium, Lavender, Rosemary, Sandalwood Patchouli.

HANGOVER – Fennel, Juniper.

HEADACHES – Lavender, Peppermint, Ho Leaf.

HYPERTENSION – Lavender, Ylang Ylang, Neroli.

HYPOTENSION – Rosemary, Peppermint.

INDIGESTION – Lavender, Fennel, Peppermint.

IMMUNE SYSTEM – Bergamot, Tea Tree, Lavender.

INFECTION – Chamomile (Roman), Tea Tree, Lavender.

INSOMNIA – Lavender, Neroli, Melissa, Rose.

MENSTRUAL PAIN – Chamomile (Roman), Clary Sage, Geranium.

MOUTH ULCERS – Tea Tree, Myrrh.

NAUSEA – Peppermint, Ginger.

NERVOUS TENSION – Marjoram, Orange, Ylang Ylang, Patchouli, Petitgrain.

PSORIASIS – Bergamot, Chamomile (Roman), Cajuput.

RASHES – Lavender.

RINGWORM – Tea Tree.

SCARS – Lavender, Neroli.

SINUSITIS – Benzoin, Cajuput, Tea Tree, Rosemary, Eucalyptus, Lemon, Ho Leaf.

SORE THROAT – Tea Tree, Sandalwood.

SPOTS – Tea Tree, Lavender.

STRESS – Lavender, Ylang Ylang, Vetiver, Neroli.

STRETCHMARKS – Mandarin, Lavender, Neroli, Lemongrass.

SUNBURN – Lavender, Tea Tree.

TOOTHACHE – Tea Tree, Lavender.

THRUSH – Tea Tree, Lavender.

VARICOSE VEINS – Geranium, Cypress, Lavender.

VERRUCAS – Tea Tree, Lemon.

WARTS – Tea Tree, Lemon.

10 | Recipes for Using Essential Oils

For minor cuts and abrasions, burns, bites and stings, essential oils are gentle, antiseptic and healing. Essential oils are good for treating colds, flu and many other conditions.

These recipes use a selection of the essential oils suitable for each condition. However, you may substitute others from the list recommended.

ACNE – A regular cleansing regime should be adopted. Steaming the affected area with Bergamot, Lavender and Tea Tree once a week will relieve congested skin. A compress of Lavender and Patchouli should be applied each evening. Lavender, Geranium and Tea Tree should be added to an oil-free, lanolin-free emollient base to protect and heal the skin. Tea Tree and Lavender may be applied directly to infected areas. As skin condition improves Lavender may be added to Jojoba and Wheatgerm and massaged to stimulate cellular function and heal scar tissue. Avoid massage where skin is infected.

ACHING MUSCLES – Add Lemongrass and Rosemary to the bath after exercise to soothe aching muscles. Massage with 2 drops Tea Tree and 2 drops Rosemary in 10mls Hazelnut oil.

ARTHRITIS – Add Chamomile (Roman), and Lavender to a bath. Gently apply 1 drop Lavender and 1 drop Peppermint in 10mls Olive oil to affected areas.

ATHLETES FOOT – Tea Tree and Lavender added to a footbath. Tea Tree applied directly to the affected areas. Patchouli and Lavender added to a footbath will aid healing of broken skin.

BRUISES – Make a compress using 1 drop Rosemary and 1 drop Lavender. Apply to the affected area. Renew as required.

BOILS – Make a compress using 1 drop Lavender and 1 Clary Sage. Apply Tea Tree to the affected area.

BROKEN CAPILLARIES – Gently apply 1 drop Geranium and 1 drop Lemon in 5ml Evening Primrose oil.

CHILBLAINS – Geranium and Lavender added to a footbath. Massage the areas with 1 drop Geranium and 1 drop Marjoram in 5mls Sweet Almond oil. Massage regularly to stimulate circulation.

CUTS AND ABRASIONS – Wash the area gently with water to which one drop Tea Tree or Lavender has been added. Apply Tea Tree or Lavender neat to the affected area 3 times per day until healing is complete. As well as being antiseptic, these essential oils will help skin to heal with the minimum of scarring. Add Tea Tree and Lavender to a fragrance free cream base for use as an effective antiseptic cream.

CELLULITE – Regular massage to affected areas will help to stimulate circulation and aid in the removal of toxins which cause this condition. Diet and exercise will also help. Make up an oil for massage using 2 drops Cypress, 2 drops Fennel, 2 drops Geranium, 2 drops Grapefruit, 2 drops Juniper in 25mls Hazelnut oil. Apply morning and evening after a bath to which Grapefruit, Fennel and Rosemary have been added.

COLD SORES – Apply Tea Tree neat to the affected area as soon as the condition appears. Adding Tea Tree, Bergamot and Lavender to the bath is effective in strengthening the immune system.

BITES AND STINGS – Wash the area gently with water to which a drop of Tea Tree or Lavender has been added. Remove sting. Apply a cold compress to which Basil and Tea Tree have been added. This should take pain and swelling away. Lavender or Tea Tree may be applied neat to the affected area 3 times per day until healing is complete.

BURNS – For minor burns, cool the affected area immediately with cold water or an ice pack. Apply Lavender neat to the area as often as required. Regular application of Lavender will aid healing and minimise scarring. Once healing is complete, massage the area with Lavender and Wheatgerm oil to speed regeneration of skin tissue and lessen scar tissue. Always remember that some skin types are prone to the formation of scar tissue and that the use of essential oils can help to lessen or even prevent this.

CATARRH – Steam inhalation with Benzoin, Eucalyptus, Cubeb. Add these essential oils to a light ring or essential oils diffuser.

COLDS AND FLU – Steam inhalation with Eucalyptus, Tea Tree and Rosemary. Bath with Bergamot, Tea Tree and Ho Leaf. Add Eucalyptus and Bergamot or Black Pepper and Cajuput to a light ring or essential oil diffuser.

DANDRUFF – Add 3 drops Tea Tree and 2 drops Cedarwood to 10mls Jojoba and massage well into the scalp. Leave on overnight. Use a gentle shampoo to remove.

DEPRESSION – Add Geranium, Ylang Ylang and Rose to a light ring or essential oil diffuser. Bath with Geranium, Clary Sage and Lime.

ECZEMA – Add Chamomile Roman to the bath. Massage affected areas with 1 drop Chamomile Roman, and 1 drop Lavender to 25ml Jojoba and Avocado oil to heal, soften and soothe irritated skin.

FATIGUE – Add Geranium and Grapefruit to the bath. Massage the body with 2 drops Geranium, 2 drops Bergamot, 2 drops Mandarin, 3 drops Vetiver to 25ml Apricot Kernel oil.

FLATULENCE – Add 1 drop Fennel and 1 drop of Mandarin or Petitgrain to 5ml Sweet Almond oil. Massage gently over abdomen and lower back. Alternatively, a compress using the same oils may be used.

FLUID RETENTION – Add Fennel to the bath. Massage the body with 2 drops Lemon, 2 drops Cypress, 2 drops Juniper, 3 drops Fennel in 20ml Hazelnut oil. Pay particular attention to dietary habits and drink plenty of pure spring water.

INSOMNIA – Add Lavender, Mandarin, Melissa and Rose to the bath. Massage the body with 2 drops Rose, 2 drops Lavender, 2 drops Neroli in 20ml Sweet Almond oil. Inhale a drop of Lavender from a tissue placed on the pillow.

NERVOUS TENSION – Add Marjoram, Orange and Ylang Ylang to the bath. Add Marjoram, Orange, Melissa to a light ring or essential oil diffuser.

PSORIASIS – Add Chamomile Roman and Bergamot to the bath. Massage the affected areas with 1 drop Bergamot, 1 drop Cajuput, to 2ml Jojoba, 5ml Avocado, and 5ml Wheatgerm oil.

SORE THROATS – Add 1 drop Tea Tree to a glass of warm water and gargle 3 times per day. Massage the throat with 1 drop Sandalwood in 5ml Jojoba morning and night.

SPOTS – For spots and problem skin Tea Tree may be applied neat to the affected area using a cotton bud. Avoid contaminating spot-free areas by using a separate cotton bud for each spot. Repeat regularly and ensure that you follow a good skincare regime and check your diet.

STRETCHMARKS – Massage affected areas twice daily with 4 drops Neroli, 3 drops Lavender, 3 drops Mandarin, in 10mls Wheatgerm and 15mls Jojoba.

STRESS – Add Ylang Ylang, Vetiver and Neroli to baths. Add Lavender, Ylang Ylang, Vetiver and Neroli to a light ring or essential oil diffuser. Inhale Vetiver and Neroli from a tissue.

SINUSITIS – For sinus problems and congestion, steam inhalation with Benzoin, Cajuput and Tea Tree and Ho Leaf, will gently and effectively relieve discomfort. Massage the sinus area using 1 drop of Cajuput in 5ml Jojoba morning and evening until the condition has diminished.

THRUSH – Lavender and Tea Tree are effective and may be added to the bath.

TOOTHACHE – Apply Tea Tree directly to affected tooth. Apply a compress of Chamomile Roman, Basil and Peppermint.

MOUTH ULCERS – Add 1 drop of Myrrh to a glass of warm water and gargle 3 times per day. Apply Tea Tree to the affected area with a cotton bud.

HEADACHES – Lavender and Peppermint are effective for treating headaches. Rub a drop of Lavender neat onto temples, or inhale from a tissue. Lavender and Peppermint used on a vaporising ring or essential oil burner are also good for relieving headaches.

NAUSEA – Peppermint inhaled from a tissue is a good remedy for nausea and is particularly effective when travelling. Ginger may also be used.

PERIODS (PAINFUL) – Apply a compress of Lavender and Clary Sage to the lower back and abdomen. Massage the lower back and abdomen with 2 drops Clary Sage and 2 drops Geranium. Add Lavender, Clary Sage and Geranium to the bath. For maximum benefit begin using these essential oils 1 week prior to menstruation.

SUNBURN – For minor sunburn, spray the area with cool spring water to which Lavender and Tea Tree essential oils have been added. Alternatively, these oils added to a cool bath are soothing and calming to overheated skin.

INSECT REPELLENT – To deter insects, add Lemongrass, Citronella or Melissa to a spray containing water. This may be sprayed onto skin or into the air. This solution could also be used to wipe down work surfaces etc. The same essential oils may be used on a vaporising ring or essential oils burner for added effect.

VARICOSE VEINS – Apply a compress of Cypress and Geranium, to affected areas. Gently apply 2 drops Lavender in 5ml Sweet Almond oil to relieve itching.

VERRUCAS – Add 1 drop Tea Tree and 1 drop Lemon to a footbath. Apply 1 drop Lemon and 1 drop Tea Tree to affected area. Cover with a plaster. Re-apply daily until condition has cleared.

WARTS – Apply 1 drop Lemon and 1 drop Tea Tree to affected area. Cover with a plaster. Re-apply daily until condition has cleared.

11 | Essential Oils and Environmental Fragrancing

To fragrance the environment and create subtle moods blend essential oils and diffuse in an essential oil vaporiser or spray into the air using a plant spray.

The essential oils can be blended according to the occasion or the season and are a pleasant and natural method of environmental fragrancing. Blend the essential oils taking into account their properties and fragrances and add to the diffuser or spray in the proportions recommended. Care must be taken to avoid polished surfaces and delicate fabrics and the skin and eyes.

Blend 2-3 drops of each oil in a clean amber glass bottle, label and use to fragrance when required.

REFRESHING – Lime, Lemon, Grapefruit, Petitgrain.

FESTIVE – Orange, Clove, Cinnamon.

HERBAL – Pine, Rosemary, Tea Tree, Eucalyptus, Ho Leaf.

FLORAL – Lavender, Geranium, Melissa.

UPLIFTING – Peppermint, Lime, Lemon.

12 | Essential Oils and Beauty Therapy

SKIN CARE

Formulate your own special skin care products using bland, unperfumed products and adding essential oils to them. You will have richly-fragrant and effective products that care for your skin naturally. Remember that you must keep to the blending proportions given and ensure that the essential oils are well blended.

In order to maintain a healthy and well-balanced skin, it is important to cleanse regularly in order to remove excess sebaceous secretions and debris which accumulate daily and may cloud the skin causing blemishes. Adopt a regime of cleansing, and toning the skin morning and night. Exfoliate the skin two or three times per week using natural scrubs to refine and remove cellular debris which will then encourage the skin to produce healthy tissue at an accelerated rate.

A face mask applied once a week will also deeply cleanse the skin and aid in the removal of impurities.

Toning the skin after cleansing or mask application will remove final traces of product and tone and refresh the skin giving a healthy glow.

Massage will relax or invigorate skin tissues according to the blend of essential oils used and also the pressure of massage strokes used and has the added benefits of toning the skin.

RECIPES

Cleansing

Add essential oils to either a cleansing milk, cleansing cream or soapless wash-off cleansing preparation. Mix well before application to the skin. Remove all cleansing preparations with either damp cotton wool pads, or sponges and warm water. Avoid using water that is too hot as this may cause excessive dryness and may cause broken capillaries. To 50mls of cleanser add up to 20 drops of essential oil. Experiment with the balance of fragrance until you find the best combination.

NORMAL SKIN – 5 drops Geranium, 5 drops Mandarin, 6 drops Clary Sage.

DRY SKIN – 5 drops Lavender, 5 drops Chamomile Roman, 6 drops Sandalwood.

SENSITIVE SKIN – 5 drops Chamomile Roman, 2 drops Melissa, 3 drops Lavender.

OILY SKIN – 5 drops Bergamot, 5 drops Tea Tree, 6 drops Ylang Ylang.

Toning

Add essential oils to spring water, put into a pump spray and shake well before spraying onto the skin to tone and refresh. To 25ml spring water, add up to 10 drops of essential oil. For extra zest use sparkling spring water and chill before spraying.

NORMAL SKIN – Geranium.

DRY SKIN – Lavender.

SENSITIVE SKIN – Chamomile Roman.

OILY SKIN – Petitgrain.

Exfoliating Scrubs

Add essential oils to a mix of natural oatmeal, bran, or ground almonds about one teaspoonful for each facial application. Two drops of essential oil. Moisten with warm water or milk to form a creamy paste. Gently apply to damp skin in small circular movements. Rinse off with warm water. Apply 2-3 times per week to keep skin looking fresh and smooth.

NORMAL SKIN – Grapefruit, Mandarin.

DRY SKIN – Rose, Sandalwood.

SENSITIVE SKIN – Chamomile Roman, Lavender.

OILY SKIN – Lemon, Tea Tree.

Masks

Natural clays are perfect for absorbing excess sebaceous secretions and cellular debris from the skin to give a more refined texture to the skin while helping to regulate the skin's ability to nourish and hydrate itself. Fuller's earth or Kaolin may be used alone or combined to formulate a base for a clay mask. A tablespoon of natural clay to which two drops of essential oil are added should be mixed to a creamy paste with warm water. Apply to the face and neck avoiding the eye area. Allow to dry and remove with warm water and sponges. To make a creamier mask which will not tighten and set on the skin, add a teaspoonful of honey, sweet almond oil or natural yoghurt to the clay mixture.

NORMAL SKIN – Geranium.

DRY SKIN – Rose.

SENSITIVE SKIN – Chamomile Roman.

OILY SKIN – Bergamot.

COMBINATION SKIN – Mix the masks to suit each skin type and apply to individual areas as required.

STIMULATING MASK FOR SALLOW SKIN – Add 1 drop each of peppermint and lemon to pep up skin circulation and brighten sallow skin.

Moisturiser

A vital part of everyday skin care, moisturisers help to seal moisture into the skin and form a protective barrier which helps prevent dehydration and cushion the skin against grime and pollution. Choose an unperfumed moisture cream or lotion for normal, dry or sensitive skin or an oil-free formulation for oily, problem skins which still require moisture but not oil. Ensure that essential oils are well-mixed before use. To 50ml of moisturiser add up to 20 drops of essential oil.

NORMAL SKIN – 4 drops Lavender, 5 drops Geranium, 6 drops Vetiver.

DRY SKIN – 4 drops Lavender, 5 drops Chamomile (Roman), 6 drops Frankincense.

SENSITIVE SKIN – 3 drops Mandarin, 4 drops Neroli, 4 drops Sandalwood.

OILY SKIN – 4 drops Bergamot, 5 drops Lavender, 6 drops Ylang Ylang.

BODY CARE

Bath and Shower Preparations

Choose unperfumed, uncoloured bath or shower gels and add essential oils to suit your skin type and your mood. Ensure that essential oils are mixed thoroughly before use.

INVIGORATE – Grapefruit, Tea Tree, Lemongrass, Juniper.

RELAX – Lavender, Clary Sage, Mandarin, Vetiver.

AFTER SPORTS – Rosemary, Lemongrass, Cypress.

ANTI-CELLULITE – Grapefruit, Lemon, Juniper, Peppermint, Fennel.

SKIN SOOTHER – Neroli, Frankincense, Melissa.

BLEMISH BANISHER – Tea Tree, Eucalyptus, Lavender, Basil, Lemon.

APHRODISIAC – Jasmine, Rose, Neroli.

MASCULINE MIX – Rosemary, Lime, Vetiver.

GENTLEMAN'S – Lime, Patchouli, Grapefriut.

PAMPER PLUS – Neroli, Geranium, Petitgrain.

CHILDREN – Lavender, Roman Chamomile, Tea Tree.

Body Exfoliators

To invigorate and stimulate the circulation while smoothing and refining skin texture, use a body exfoliating scrub daily on all but the most sensitive skin to dramatically improve the appearance of the skin. Apply to damp skin using a loofah or flannel mitt in sweeping circular strokes. Rinse off with warm water. Pat skin dry. Use regularly to ensure smooth healthy skin. Body exfoliators should be used prior to the application of massage oils or skin preparations as they prepare the skin and allow for the maximum penetration of essential oils.

Add essential oils to 2 tablespoons of oatmeal mixed with 2 tablespoons of salt, mix to a creamy paste with warm water. Add 1 drop of each essential oil and blend well.

INVIGORATOR. – Peppermint, Grapefruit, Bergamot.

SMOOTHER – Rose, Geranium, Sandalwood.

GENTLEMEN'S – Rosemary, Cypress, Eucalyptus.

CELLULITE – Fennel, Grapefruit, Lime.

TONING – Petitgrain, Lemongrass, Cedarwood.

CHILDREN – Lavender, Roman Chamomile, Tea Tree.

Lotions

An important part of any bodycare regime, body lotions enrich and protect the skin keeping it soft and healthy whilst imparting an all-over feeling of wellbeing. Use after every bath or shower and apply generously to all areas especially feet, knees and elbows which tend to be extra dry. To 100ml of body lotion add up to 40 drops of essential oil.

Add essential oils to unperfumed body lotion or cream according to preference.

RECIPES

ENRICHED – 12 drops Clary Sage, 10 drops Orange, 15 drops Frankincense.

GENTLEMAN'S – 12 drops Marjoram, 10 drops Lime, 15 drops Vetiver.

LUXURY – 12 drops Rose, 10 drops Melissa, 15 drops Benzoin.

ALL PURPOSE – 12 drops Lavender, 10 drops Mandarin, 15 drops Bergamot.

SPORTY – 12 drops Basil, 10 drops Rosemary, 15 drops Lemongrass.

SPICE – 12 drops Cypress, 10 drops Benzoin, 15 drops Frankincense.

EXOTIC – 12 drops Black Pepper, 10 drops Orange, 15 drops Geranium.

CHILDREN – 5 drops Lavender, 5 drops Roman Chamomile, 5 drops Tea Tree.

Hand and Foot Care
Hands and feet are often much neglected and can become rough and dry. Pamper and care for hands and feet by regular soaks in warm fragrant essential oil baths, and exfoliating scrubs to smooth away hard skin. Follow with the application of rich emollient preparations and you will be amazed at how good hands and feet will soon look and feel. To 25ml of cream, add up to 10 drops of essential oil.

RECIPES

Hand or Foot Soaks
Add 4 drops of essential oils to warm soapy water, agitate well and relax.

ANTISEPTIC AND HEALING –
Lavender, Lemon, Tea Tree.
Lavender, Geranium, Benzoin.
Bergamot, Tea Tree, Cajuput.
Patchouli, Lavender, Lemon.

Hand and Foot Creams

SOOTHING AND ENRICHED –

3 drops Lavender, 3 drops Mandarin, 4 drops Sandalwood.
3 drops Rose, 3 drops Melissa, 4 drops Petitgrain.
3 drops Lime, 3 drops Clary Sage, 4 drops Frankincense.
3 drops Neroli, 3 drops Chamomile (Roman) 4 drops Geranium.

For a luxurious foot treatment, soak the feet for 10-15 minutes. Use an exfoliating scrub; massage your favourite soothing enriched cream well into the feet and cover with a pair of cotton socks. Leave overnight to allow the essential oils to penetrate and soften the skin. Apply this treatment regularly for beautifully soft feet.

For a luxurious hand treatment follow a similar procedure with the hands and apply cotton gloves overnight. Regular treatment in this manner will improve and maintain the condition of the hands.

HAIRCARE

To impart a delicate fragrance and enhance body and shine whilst treating your hair gently and naturally, add essential oils to unperfumed shampoos and conditioners and use regularly to maintain beautiful hair and a healthy scalp. Constant use of essential oils together with massage to the scalp can have a stimulating effect on the scalp which may be helpful in nourishing and feeding the hair follicles to promote new hair growth.

For a deep acting treatment to condition and strengthen the hair use Jojoba with your choice of essential oils once every week and leave overnight to act on the hair and scalp. Add shampoo to the hair and massage well before rinsing thoroughly with warm water.

Avoid over washing the hair as this will strip natural oils and leave hair weak and damaged.

RECIPES

Shampoo

Add essential oils to your favourite mild cleansing shampoo. Use regularly for best effect. Always rinse with clear water to remove any residues.

NORMAL HAIR – Lavender, Grapefruit, Geranium.

DRY HAIR – Sandalwood, Ylang Ylang, Chamomile Roman.

OILY HAIR – Tea Tree, Peppermint, Lemon, Cedarwood.

DEEP CLEANSING – Grapefruit, Lemon, Geranium.

FAIR HAIR – Chamomile Roman.

DARK HAIR – Rosemary, Patchouli.

Conditioners

Apply after each shampoo, leave for a couple of minutes then rinse thoroughly with clear water. To 30ml shampoo, add essential oils and mix well before use.

NORMAL HAIR – 5 drops Lavender, 4 drops Rosemary, 4 drops Geranium.

DRY HAIR – 5 drops Chamomile Roman, 4 drops Sandalwood, 4 drops Neroli.

OILY HAIR – 5 drops Tea Tree, 4 drops Ylang Ylang, 4 drops Grapefruit.

DANDRUFF – 5 drops Tea Tree, 4 drops Cedarwood, 4 drops Lavender.

Deep Conditioning Treatments
Apply once a week and leave on the hair overnight to nourish and deep condition the hair. Apply shampoo directly to the hair before adding water and rinsing thoroughly with warm water. Use 15 ml Jojoba and add essential oils to this before massaging well into the hair and scalp. Longer hair may require more Jojoba to cover all areas of the hair thoroughly.

NORMAL HAIR – 2 drops Lavender, 2 drops Grapefruit, 2 drops Geranium.

DRY HAIR – 2 drops Chamomile Roman, 2 drops Lavender, 2 drops Sandalwood.

OILY HAIR – 2 drops Tea Tree, 2 drops Petitgrain, 2 drops Patchouli.

THINNING OR WEAK HAIR – 2 drops Lavender, 2 drops Rosemary, 2 drops Grapefruit.

13 | Conclusion

Now that you have experienced and enjoyed the benefits of essential oils and aromatherapy I am sure that you are well aware of how useful this therapy can be to you in your everyday life. You will probably find yourself using essential oils daily and confidently, and perhaps you have even formulated recipes from your favourite essential oils! You will, no doubt, be fragranced delightfully wherever you go and will look and feel great.

I hope that you will continue to experiment and enjoy the benefits of this natural aromatic therapy.

14 | Further Reading and Information

Aromatherapy – Micheline Arcier. Hamlyn.

The Art of Aromatherapy – Robert Tisserand. C.W. Daniel.

Aromatherapy – A Guide for Home Use – Christine Westwood. Amberwood.

Aromatherapy – A Nurse's Guide – Ann Percival. Amberwood.

Essential Oils in Colour – Rosemary Caddy. Amberwood.

If you require a professional aromatherapist, the organisations listed below will be able to supply you with a list of their members in your area. These aromatherapists have undergone a thorough and rigorous training in all aspects of the subject and the professional bodies to which they belong ensure that a high standard of treatment will be offered to clients by constantly monitoring and setting safety standards.

Federation of Holistic Therapists
38a Portsmouth Road
Woolston
Southampton
Hampshire SO2 9AD.

International Federation of Aromatherapists
Dept. of Continuing Education
The Royal Masonic Hospital
Ravenscourt Park
London W6 0TN.

OTHER BOOKS FROM AMBERWOOD PUBLISHING ARE:

Aromatherapy Lexicon – The Essential Reference by Geoff Lyth and Sue Charles is a colourful, fun way to learn about Aromatherapy. £4.99.

Aromatherapy – The Baby Book by Marion Del Gaudio Mak. An easy to follow guide to massage for the infant or child. £3.99

Aromatherapy – A Guide for Home Use by Christine Westwood. All you need to know about essential oils and using them. £1.99.

Aromatherapy – for Stress Management by Christine Westwood. Covering the use of essential oils for everyday stress-related problems. £3.50.

Aromatherapy – For Healthy Legs and Feet by Christine Westwood. A guide to the use of essential oils for the treatment of legs and feet. £2.99.

Aromatherapy – The Pregnancy Book by Jennie Supper RM RN MGCP. Jennie Supper, a State Registered Nurse and Midwife explains the use of Aromatherapy during pregnancy and the common conditions which may be treated safely. £5.99

Aromatherapy – A Nurses Guide by Ann Percival SRN. The ultimate, safe, lay guide to the natural benefits of Aromatherapy. Including recipes and massage techniques for many medical conditions and a quick reference chart. £2.99.

Aromatherapy – A Nurses Guide for Women by Ann Percival SRN. Concentrates on women's health for all ages. Including sections on PMT, menopause, infertility, cellulite. £2.99.

Aromatherapy – Essential Oils in Colour by Rosemary Caddy Bsc Hons, ARCS MISP is a unique book depicting the chemistry of essential oils. £9.99.

Aroma Science – The Chemistry & Bioactivity of Essential Oils by Dr Maria Lis-Balchin. With a comprehensive list of the Oils and scientific analysis. Includes sections on the sense of smell and the history of Aromatherapy. £5.99.

Woman Medicine – Vitex Agnus Castus by Simon Mills MA, FNIMH. The story of the herb that has been used for centuries in the treatment of women's problems. £2.99.

Plant Medicine – A Guide for Home Use (New Edition) by Charlotte Mitchell MNIMH. A guide to home use giving an insight into the wonderful healing qualities of plants. £2.99.

Feng Shui – A Guide for Home use by Karen Ward. Simple tips on "Power of Place" and effects of environment of health. £2.99

Ancient Medicine – Ginkgo Biloba (New Edition) by Dr Desmond Corrigan BSc(Pharms), MA, Phd, FLS, FPSI. Improved memory, circulation and concentration are associated with Ginkgo and explained in this book. £2.99.

Indian Medicine – The Immune System by Dr Desmond Corrigan BSc(Pharms), MA, Phd, FLS, FPSI. An intriguing account of the history of the plant called Echinacea and its power to influence the immune system. £2.99.

Herbal Medicine for Sleep & Relaxation by Dr Desmond Corrigan BSc(Pharms), MA, PhD, FLS, FPSI. A guide to the natural sedatives as an alternative to orthodox drug therapies, drawing on the latest medical research, presented in an easy reference format. £2.99.

Herbal First Aid by Andrew Chevallier BA, MNIMH. A beautifully clear reference book of natural remedies and general first aid in the home. £3.50.

Natural Taste – Herbal Teas, A Guide for Home Use by Andrew Chevallier BA, MNIMH. Contains a comprehensive compendium of Herbal Teas gives information on how to make it, its benefits, history and folklore. £3.50.

Garlic– How Garlic Protects Your Heart by Prof E. Ernst MD, PhD. Used as a medicine for over 4500 years, this book examines the latest scientific evidence supporting Garlic's effect in reducing cardiovascular disease, the Western World's number one killer. £3.99.

Phytotherapy – Fifty Vital Herbs by Andrew Chevallier, the most popular medicinal herbs with uses and advice written by an expert. £6.99

Insomnia – Doctor I Can't Sleep by Dr Adrian Williams FRCP. Written by one of the world's leading sleep experts, Dr Williams explains the phenomenon of sleep and sleeping disorders and gives advice on treatment. With 25% of the adult population reporting difficulties sleeping – this book will be essential reading for many. £2.99.

Eyecare Eyewear – For Better Vision by Mark Rossi Bsc, MBCO. A complete guide to eyecare and eyewear including an assessment of the types of spectacles and contact lenses available and the latest corrective surgical procedures. £3.99.

Arthritis and Rheumatism by Dr John Cosh FRCP, MD. Covers all forms of Arthritis, its effects and the treatments available. £4.95.

All You Ever Wanted To Know About Vitamins by Dr Leonard Mervyn. The ultimate book on nutrition. £6.99.